COMMON SENSE WEIGHT CONTROL

by

Benjamin D. Gordon, M.D.

Common Sense Weight Control
by Benjamin D. Gordon, M.D.

Copyright 2012 Benjamin D. Gordon, M.D.
Smashwords Edition

Digital edition created by GoPublished
www.gopublished.com

TABLE OF CONTENTS

I NEVER PUT MY PATIENTS ON A DIET!

The word "diet" is understood by everyone's subconscious mind as "deprivation" ---- "I'm not going to be able to eat the things I like" which is the same as saying to yourself "I have to be punished" ---- "I'm bad" ---- "There's something wrong with me".

That's a terrible thing to tell anyone. Two things are important to know:

1) The body has natural responses to outside influences. For example, if you drink a lot of water, your glands will make your kidneys pass more water to keep the body in balance.

And it's the same with food. If you suddenly give the body less than it's used to getting, your metabolism adapts by slowing down to save energy. The body will do whatever has to be done to keep working normally. It responds to the decreased food supply.

Fat is stored energy. When fat stores are lost quickly, as with drastic "no fat" diets, the body responds by making an enzyme whose function is to replace those fat stores as quickly as possible as soon as it gets regular food again. That's why people who lose weight quickly gain it back so fast. The body is trying to preserve and protect its "energy storage supply". This is a metabolic process, millions of years old, that allowed humans to survive.

(2) There are genetic differences between people.

Some have a naturally high metabolic rate, a high energy level and they burn up most of the calories in the food they eat. We all know those who can eat steaks, French fries, banana splits and milk shakes but never gain weight.

The other extreme are those who eat one piece of pie and gain. Actually, evidence now shows that those people have a very efficient metabolism. They handle the food so well there are left-over calories that can go "into storage".

Most of us fall somewhere in between. That's why I prefer to teach my patients the basic principles of weight management and allow *them* to be in control. Each person will figure out how to use this information in a way that is most comfortable for him or her.

THREE MAIN PRINCIPLES

There are three main principles:

A. Reducing the fat content of what you eat and learning where there is "hidden fat"; i.e., fat of which you are not aware.

For example, chocolate is usually milk chocolate, with milk fats. Most people just think of the "sweet". Pasta is not that fattening, especially if you buy whole wheat pasta. It's the oil and meat in the sauce. Just put on less sauce and mix it more thoroughly. This way you're not deprived. You get the flavor of the sauce but avoid the excess. We all know what happens when we put on a lot of sauce: we reach for the bread to wipe it up. Once you're aware of this, you can avoid the extra calories and yet not feel deprived.

Fact: When the body burns carbohydrate or protein, it gets 4 calories /gram but fat gives 9 calories /gram. You don't want to eliminate fat completely because some vitamins are fat-soluble and are absorbed with the fat. Reducing the amount can help with weight control. Start reading the nutritional labels on everything. For example, there is one spaghetti sauce with no fat, one with one gram/ounce and others with 3 – 7 grams /ounce. Knowing this gives you control over what you pick. With packages of "Low Moisture Skim Milk Mozzarella", two brands have no fat while others may have up to 6 grams. Knowledge gives you control.

Look at every food you eat and think of how it's made. Pies, pastries, cake, cookies, donuts, Danish and muffins are made with oil, shortening, butter or margarine and milk. But if, one day, you say "I haven't had a muffin in a month. I want one today." --- have one. You haven't eaten it because YOU decided not to, not because a "diet" imposed the restriction on you. You won't feel deprived since YOU are in control.

Some foods with fat content are obvious: French fries, potato chips, many snacks, luncheon meats (bologna, salami) are loaded with fat, --- but you can buy fat-free bologna. Raw vegetables in a salad are great but find a fat-free dressing you like --- or use less of the regular dressing. In a restaurant, I often ask for wedges of lemon to squeeze on the salad. Use lemon or herbs on fish, not breading (which usually has oil) or cream sauce. On a baked potato, just use less butter or sour cream. Just control the excess. Peanut butter has 16 -17 grams of fat per ounce. Spread it on thinly. Have it in the morning when you'll be active all day. Don't make this an evening snack. Obviously, don't have any snack before bed. Metabolism lowers when you sleep so unused calories go into "storage".

Go heavily on fresh fruits, vegetables (raw or cooked) and whole grains (non-sugared cereal, whole wheat pasta or bread). Many people say they don't like raw veggies (broccoli, cauliflower, carrots, string beans, radishes, cucumbers, etc.). One thing we all know is that food tastes best when you're very hungry. That's the time to take a raw vegetable or fruit when you're looking for a snack. You'll discover what led man to find these foods in nature thousands of years ago --- when he was hungry.

As you start opening your mind to possibilities, you'll discover all sorts of things. I've learned this from listening to patients. The traditional way to make tuna salad is with mayonnaise. There are fat-free varieties of this which can be combined with mustard or ketchup, fat-free salad dressing or yogurt with herbs, tomatoes, green peppers or celery.

B An Exercise Program

There is no way you can control your weight without this. The evidence for the beneficial effects of exercise (ideally 5 times a week) is overwhelming. A combination of aerobics and weight training is important:

> a) Aerobic exercise (walking, running, bicycling) uses calories while you're active and builds your stamina.

b) Proper weight training builds muscle, even in the elderly, and muscle continues to burn calories after you've stopped the workout. If you're out of condition, *start slowly and carefully*, no matter how much of an athlete you were or in what condition you had been.

What does "being in condition" really mean? Your lungs don't change size. The amount of air you breathe is not that different. What happens?

Your body's metabolism and physiology change as you exercise day by day so that the oxygen you do breathe in begins to be used *more efficiently* by the cells of your muscles and blood vessels. That's why you get your "second wind". When you're "in condition", your body uses oxygen more effectively.

One way this happens relates to the endothelium (the inner lining) of your blood vessels. These cells produce two substances:

one widens and one narrows the arteries as needed by your body activities. A study done at the University of Pisa in Italy suggests that exercise can protect the endothelium from age-related deterioration. In athletic 60 year olds, it was as functional as those in their thirties.

Most interesting was finding that it's never too late to start. Even in people with known coronary artery disease, exercise improved their endothelial function.

Studies in homes for the elderly have shown that properly supervised weight training allows even frail 90 years olds to get out of chairs more easily and move around with an improved sense of well-being and stability.

An important point about using weights is knowing the difference between training and straining. When someone lifts too much to "see if he can" or to show off, muscles and tendons get torn, ligaments get strained and the result is weakness, not strength. Strength is built by lifting small weights, that are comfortable for you, in sets of repetitions (6 or 10 or 12 times), resting, and then doing one or two more sets. Different movements strengthen different muscles. Knowing what to do is important. Supervision by a trained professional is advisable when you start. Learning how to use equipment properly, and how to progress, will keep you safe as well as make you strong.

There are many good fitness counselors and excellent exercise videos available. However, you don't always need special equipment. You can lie on the floor and do pelvic tilts, leg raises, head raises, push ups - - but always start slowly with what you can do easily, and then build up gradually.

Running in place is still a great aerobic exercise. Years ago, when I was busy with my medical practice, I didn't exercise for some time. When I decided to "get back into shape", I began to run in place. I was shocked to find I couldn't go more than 20 seconds. However, I continued every day. After a week, I could last a minute. After two weeks, almost 5 minutes. In the third week, I found my "second wind" and was pleasantly surprised to find 10 minutes was not a problem. Now at 84, and after two hip replacements which restrict running, walking on a treadmill or an elliptical unit, an exercise bicycle and weight training do very well. If I get busy and don't exercise, it's nice to find that two or three weeks will bring back energy and a feeling of "well-being".

Obviously, if you have any medical problem, beginning an exercise program should be discussed with a physician.

C Water

I never ask people to drink a certain number of glasses a day. When we're drinking, we all know when we've had enough. Our body tells us that. After brushing your teeth in the morning, drink ½ - 2 glasses. If you take pills of any kind, always drink at least ½ - 1 glass with them. This usually prevents stomach irritation from the medication.

Don't pass up a drinking fountain or a sink. Naturally, stop the water intake after 7:00 PM so you won't do nighttime toilet trekking.

Why the water?

When you exercise and control calorie intake, your fat stores break down. These breakdown products come into your bloodstream and are passed out of your body through the kidneys into your urine. They are not very soluble, like salts, and require a lot of water to wash them out. If they are not washed out, they combine back into fat. People ask about other liquids. Tea and diet sodas are OK; not sweet or cola drinks. They are just adding extra calories back. Plain water is best.

There are some traps which can interfere with these methods of weight control.

One trap is failure to eat breakfast. The body's metabolism responds to the type and amount of food and water it gets. Just juice and coffee in the morning gets the body to respond by slowing down. It's preparing to be starved. Lunch is usually not a major meal, but watch the fats that can be there. If you've eaten little during the day and are then hungry in the evening, a big dinner on a slow metabolism when you'll be resting and sleeping later leaves unburned calories to be "stored".

A good breakfast does many things. First, by providing a lot of food, it "revs up" the metabolic rate because there's "a lot to handle". Secondly, it sets you up for better functioning during the day. Our brain is the only part of our body whose cells use carbohydrate exclusively as their source of energy. Cereals, whole grain bread, wheat germ and unprocessed bran are among the best sources of the B vitamins. B vitamins help metabolize carbohydrate. Eaten in the morning, it helps your brain work better and gives you energy. Children who eat a good breakfast (no sugared cereals) do better in school. A dish of whole grain cereal (90 – 120 calories to the ounce) provides a good way to introduce fruits into your diet, even several at a time: bananas, strawberries, blueberries, peaches, prunes, blackberries, raspberries, etc. Add a tablespoon of wheat germ or bran for extra vitamin B. As a variation from skim or low-fat milk, many of my patients use juice on their cereal --- cranberry, apple, prune, orange, grapefruit --- or whatever you like. A citrus fruit or juice, cereal with more fruits, whole grain bread with butter or margarine (OK at the start of the day) and a beverage makes an appropriate and nourishing breakfast. Pancakes or waffles with a reduced-calorie syrup can be an alternative. Years ago, the Harvard Heart Letter described research data showing that fiber could reduce heart disease risk. They studied over 68,000 women for 10 years and found those eating the most fiber, especially cereal fiber, had less coronary heart disease.

Eggs have been badly maligned for years. The profession is now beginning to appreciate the fact that the yolk is nature's food source for a new developing life. It is a source of balanced nutrition with nutrients common to many species. It has cholesterol and also anti-cholesterol factors. It has iron, lecithin, calcium, protein and is one of the very few natural food sources of vitamin D. D helps the body to absorb calcium, which is why it was added to milk years ago in the days when there were children with rickets. As adults, we're not out in sunshine as much as when we were children so this provides extra D. If you are allergic to eggs, you can take Cod Liver Oil capsules, which also have vitamin A, essential fatty acids and fish oils. Vitamin D is especially important for post-menopausal women to help them absorb calcium. Since vitamins A, D and E are stored in the body's fat, it is possible to overdose on them. Ask your doctor or pharmacist if you have any questions about what you're already taking.

Another trap is our society's habit of snacking; e.g., coffee and Danish mid-morning, candy bars, ice cream, sandwiches with luncheon meats, etc. With calories supplied every few hours, there's no need to draw on the body's "storage supply". If you must snack, use fruit or raw vegetables. Too many times, children who want a snack are given a "sweet" (a cookie or lollipop) and become conditioned to this taste when hungry. One patient, who'd been heavy as a child, vowed her children would not have to go through the weight-losing battle she'd had. When hungry, she'd give them a raw vegetable – celery with cream cheese, a slice of plain cheese, fresh fruit – real food. When they were old enough to go to birthday parties, they didn't care for the sweets. They could take them or leave them. They were never obsessed by them.

One man, returning for his annual exam, had lost 30 lbs. I asked "Tell me what you really did". He answered "I did what you suggested. I reduced the amount of fat in my diet. I began to eat a good breakfast. I started an exercise routine and drank a lot of water. For dinner, I ate nothing but fresh fruit. I ate as much as I wanted so I wouldn't be hungry, but just the fruit".

Now it was my turn to learn. Though this

would not satisfy most people, I realized the importance of a low-fat meal in the evening. Vegetables (no butter sauce), brown rice (as little butter or oil as possible), small chunks of lean meat, skinless poultry, fish or seafood occasionally in some whole wheat pasta would work well, too. Dessert could be fat-free frozen yoghurt, fat-free cake or fresh fruit. I think his fruit meals worked so well due to the water content. Obviously, there will be times when you may go out to eat socially or there are family gatherings and strict adherence will not be possible. Just go back to your regular routine the next day. There's no need to feel that you've "failed".

Years ago, the Tufts University Health and Nutrition Letter described the Dallas cowboys as one of the healthiest professional sports teams. They had changed the "meat" concept and were now big on broccoli, cauliflower, carrots, bananas and oranges. Meat was not eliminated completely but was used in proper proportion.

All the principles described here are based on recommendations of professional nutritionists. As I've listened to "food fads" during the years, the best thinking seems to come back around to a well-balanced diet supplied by the basic food groups with special emphasis on fruits, vegetables and whole grains. Doing things this way, when, how and what you eat is under your control because you have taken command. Thus, the final victory belongs to you alone -- and you'll be in shape to make mischief.

www.ingramcontent.com/pod-product-compliance
Lightning Source LLC
Chambersburg PA
CBHW050801250726
48662CB00005B/2339